I'm Ju[...]Me

Claudia

Always share your thoughts

Mary

Fallcon 2022

I'm Just Me

A Life with Turner Syndrome & Nonverbal Learning Disorder

Mary Yoakum

Yoakum Enterprises, LLC
Denver, Colorado

I'm Just Me: A Life with Turner Syndrome
and Nonverbal Learning Disorder
Mary Yoakum
Copyright © 2022 by Mary Yoakum

ISBN, Print Version: 979-8-9865820-0-9
ISBN, Electronic Version: 979-8-9865820-1-6
LCCN: 2022912839

Yoakum Enterprises, LLC
Denver, Colorado

Editing by Melanie Mulhall, Dragonheart
Cover and interior design by Bob Schram, Bookends Design

First Edition
Printed in the United States of America

Dedicated to the friends and families
of women with Turner Syndrome
to facilitate understanding and communication

Contents

Foreword

I WAS FIRST APPROACHED by Mary pre-pandemic about her desire to document her development and life to inform and educate other girls and women with Turner Syndrome (TS) and nonverbal learning disorder (NLD). We met to discuss the progress on the book at several national conferences and connected numerous times over the telephone and video meetings regarding the content, sequence, and scope of the book. Mary's hard work over the past few years has resulted in a book that lets the reader experience the day-to-day triumphs and hardships of a woman with TS and NLD. We get a glimpse of how women with TS perceive themselves and how others in the neurotypical community perceive them.

Mary demonstrates a deep understanding of TS and NLD with meaningful examples, and she puts into everyday terms what many clinicians and researchers like me theorize. Each chapter deals with a specific topic pertinent to most women and girls with TS and NLD in an understanding, supportive, and even humorous way. Lessons are summarized at the end of each chapter.

Mary gives parents ideas on how to respond to their daughters with TS and how to address the struggles within the family and in the community. This book tackles difficult subjects like bullying, meltdowns, and social, educational, and vocational challenges. She also makes suggestions for parents about how to navigate the educational maze by advocating for their child.

Mary's book speaks to each of us personally and teaches those with TS how to develop their own internal rudder (one of Mary's unique concepts) and how the rest of us need to let them take control of the rudder.

To the girls and women with TS, as Mary would say, take control. Stop floating down the river aimlessly and start steering your life in the direction you desire.

–DR. DEAN MOONEY
July 2022

Introduction

WE ALL HAVE STRENGTHS AND WEAKNESSES. We all have challenges to overcome. But in the end, I am just me, like you are just you.

When I talk about who I am, I have to talk about Turner Syndrome (TS). The problem is that when I do that, I can literally see the light change in the other person's eyes, and they start treating me differently. That's why I have a hard time telling anyone about TS. It's also why now, in my sixties, I am just starting to come to terms with Turner Syndrome and learning to accept it.

If you are a parent of a child with Turner Syndrome, be an involved parent and ask questions. There are too many issues for any child, let alone one with TS, to cope with alone. They will need your help.

Turner Syndrome is a genetic disorder found only in females. Normally, humans have forty-six chromosomes in each cell, and among those forty-six chromosomes are two X chromosomes for females. But with Turner Syndrome, there is either a missing X chromosome or one regular X chromosome and one broken X chromosome. This can cause a lot of health and learning issues. One of these learning issues for many girls with TS is nonverbal learning disorder (NLD).

Even with all these challenges, we can learn to lead independent and fulfilling lives. We just need extra time and effort to get to where we need to be. My desire with this guide is to provide the parents of girls with Turner Syndrome (and the health issues related to it) a bit of gentle guidance from one who has experienced TS from the inside-out, has a few stories to tell about her experience, and can offer a lesson or two to assist you in helping your daughter.

CHAPTER 1

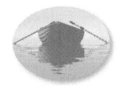

Lather, Rinse, Repeat

IMAGINE THAT YOU ARE TALKING to someone using the same language, but you can't comprehend what they are saying. Your neurons and synapses aren't sending information that processes the meaning of what is being said in the same way they do for those without Turner Syndrome and nonverbal learning disorder. Throw in hearing and vision impairment and that is me.

Let me give you an example. I was having a telephone conversation with one of my brothers about a trip I'd taken to Mexico, and I said I felt I'd bought out the stores. He replied, "Oh. Then I guess I won't go there for a while."

Everything just froze in place. I couldn't understand why he couldn't go. Then he repeated what he'd said, and it clicked. He was being humorous. If I'd bought the shops out, then he would have to wait until the vendors replaced their stock before he could buy anything. This need for many of us with TS to hear what is being said more than once to be able to understand it fully is something I often humorously refer to as lather, rinse, repeat. To get the full meaning of what is being said, we need repetition.

What I have just described is a cognitive processing and functioning issue. And it not only impacts what I hear, but also what I say. More than others, it's important for me to think before I speak. If it's important, like a meeting with my boss, I need to take a minute to think about the information I'm about to impart, including what the other person knows and what they need to know about the subject of the conversation.

Then I think about how to organize what I'm going to say to ensure that I provide information in a logical, sequential way.

Sometimes when I'm speaking on a subject, I start at the beginning and then leapfrog, skipping important information. In those cases, the person I'm talking with often stops me and asks me to back up and fill in the blanks. Thinking about what I need to say before I say it—essentially mapping it out—can help me avoid that problem.

Of course, a person cannot always plan out what they're going to say. If I'm stopped in a hallway and asked a question off the cuff, I may have difficulty with that. If I can plan it out, I'm good, but if it's extemporaneous, I may be in trouble.

For instance, as a member of Toastmasters International, I can give a speech without problems because I have the opportunity to plan it out in advance. But if I participate in a Toastmasters table topics session, I'm likely going to struggle because table topics are meant to help members improve their ability to handle impromptu speaking. And that is not my strong suit.

The majority of those with Turner Syndrome also have hearing problems, which impacts our ability to understand and communicate with others. Hearing aides are beneficial, but they don't correct the hearing problems like glasses correct vision problems They simply make things louder so the wearer can more easily hear what is being said. And hearing aids don't come without challenges. For instance, background noises (other people talking, ambient sounds, music) can make it difficult to hear and understand what others are saying to you and can even be painful to the ears.

When I was a child, my school nurse told my mother I had difficulty hearing, so I was taken to a hearing specialist when I was ten. The specialist tested my hearing and confirmed that I had a hearing deficiency. I saw the same specialist again when I was seventeen and twenty-one, but I never got hearing aids. My mother died when I was twenty-five, and I was working a minimum wage job at the time. I couldn't afford to buy hearing aids, and I did not have insurance to pay for them. I finally got a pair in my forties, but they were not the right type for my specific hearing loss and were problematic to work with, so I didn't wear them. Finally, when I was fifty-six and had the help of both my employer and the state Division of Vocational Rehabilitation, I was able to get hearing aids that actually worked for me. I wear them constantly, and the clinic through which I got them follows up with me once a year and adjusts them as needed.

Because a high percentage of Turner Syndrome girls have hearing problems, their hearing should be tested regularly. Your pediatrician can help you select a hearing specialist or the Turner Syndrome Society of the United States can help you find a local TS clinic, and they can help you find a hearing specialist.

These are some of the things girls with Turner Syndrome must deal with. And because nonverbal learning disorder is an important part of it, I'm going to talk about that next.

• **Lesson 1:** *Because of the way we process information cognitively and because we often have hearing deficits, you will probably have to repeat yourself. You may find this frustrating, but that is the way we work. We are not being difficult or insolent. We are just trying to understand and communicate with you.*

• **Lesson 2:** *Know that because we have issues with cognitive processing, we also need an opportunity to think before we are asked to speak and that this will impact how we handle unexpected and impromptu conversations.*

• **Lesson 3:** *The majority of girls with Turner Syndrome also have hearing problems. Get her tested for this early and buy her hearing aids if they are needed.*

CHAPTER 2

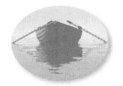

Nonverbal Learning Disorder

BECAUSE NONVERBAL LEARNING DISORDER (NLD) is
present in many girls with Turner Syndrome, it is
something to understand and be aware of. Nonverbal learning disorder is a pattern of cognitive and
neurological strengths and deficits that significantly
affect an individual's ability to learn and function
both within an academic setting and outside it in or-
dinary life. Girls with both TS and NLD have both
assets and deficits stemming from nonverbal learning
disorder.

Abilities with simple motor skills, auditory perception, and rote learning fall into the assets column.
We often develop a very good ability to listen to and

understand simple, repetitive verbal material. And we frequently have a well-developed ability to cognitively process and understand verbal language (known as receptive language skills). We can be good at memorizing material and reciting it (rote verbal ability). We're good at learning through hearing and repetition, and for that reason, we may develop a large vocabulary and have a higher level of recall than many others. This can lead us to love talking, and we often talk a lot. These positive characteristics tend to be more prominent as we age.

At the same time, we often have deficits in tactile and visual perception, spatial organization, and complex psychomotor skills. Among other things, that may mean we have trouble drawing, writing, and using analog clocks. And tasks that require motor coordination, like tying shoes, may also be a problem.

We can have trouble perceiving objects or judging sensations through the sense of touch. In other words, we have challenges with the awareness of objects in the space around us and how they fit together. Our awareness of our body's position in space can also be affected, which can make us appear clumsy. I seemed to bump into the coffee table a lot when I was young.

Some activities I've come across that can help us understand and interact with the environment better include playing with Legos and going through (age appropriate) obstacle courses. Playing with Legos helps teach us how objects fit into the world around us and obstacle courses help us understand how we move through the world.

Because of our visual perception and psychomotor issues, many women with Turner Syndrome and NLD (including me) don't drive. While I once owned a car and drove, an accident related to these issues led me to make the decision to abandon driving and use public transportation, and I've become very adept at that. And I have developed tactics for handling going to new and unfamiliar parts of town: I always take my planner and phone with me. I have the phone number of the person I'm contacting and the address of my destination in my planner, and if I get turned around, I can call and get help with directions. That really works for me.

Those with nonverbal learning disorder can have trouble learning new things—something that can worsen with age—and because of that, we can become rigid in our daily routines and interactions with others. We just seem to deal with novel material and situations poorly and sometimes inappropriately, so that rigidity is a coping mechanism.

Where new situations are concerned, I'm fine if someone can work with me on knowing the steps needed to get to the desired end result. If the steps change along the way, I can still work with them, though my stomach may clench a little. An example of this is flying. I usually try to fly nonstop, but sometimes that's not possible, either because of the destination or because the flight gets diverted. In either case, I go directly to the new gate assignment and hang out there, whether that is for a few minutes or a couple of hours. Yes, my stomach may clench a little, but being at the gate ahead of time is comforting.

Another deficit is difficulty academically with mathematics and science that requires the application of math. Reading comprehension can also be a problem, particularly if the concepts in the written material are implied but not clearly expressed or are ambiguous. And while we do like to talk, written expression can be a challenge.

Social and behavioral deficits are also associated with NLD, particularly deficits in social perception, social judgment, and social interaction skills. We may have a tendency to withdraw socially, and this tendency can be heightened as we get older, leading to social isolation. As children, we may act out (externalized behavior) or become anxious or depressed (internalized behavior). Those tendencies increase as we move from childhood into adolescence and adulthood.

The social aspects of nonverbal learning disorder can be likened to boats drifting on the river of life. How we use our boat's rudder will determine where we go and what adventures we will have. With NLD, you don't know you have a rudder and therefore don't know how to control it. Because of that, others, such as family, need to step in and assist with rudder control until you learn how to manage your own rudder.

Until a girl with NLD learns how to manage her own rudder, she will be vulnerable to the control of others.

The example I am going to give is simplistic, but I believe it will help get my point across. Picture floating down the river enjoying its sights, sounds, and basic rhythm when you notice a tree with a swing on it. You want to dock your boat so you can play on the swing, but you can't because someone else is in charge of your rudder and they won't dock the boat. You may huff and puff and cross your arms to show your displeasure with their decision, but what are you going to do? They're in charge of your rudder. You don't understand that you have the right to say, "But I want to play on the swing!" You just suck it up and soldier on.

You continue to float along and see a merry-go-round. The person in charge of your rudder says, "Let's play on the merry-go-round." You go because they control your rudder. It's okay. You have fun. It's not the swing, but it's okay because you have fun.

With nonverbal learning disorder, until we gain the maturity to understand rudders, we don't have rudder control. Think of children and how spontaneous they are. They just go and do. They have much less self-control than an adult, and it takes a lot of effort to teach them about focus and direction. In essence, they are rudderless. The parent of a girl with nonverbal learning disorder must teach their daughter that they have a rudder and how to control it. Until then, you will have to be in charge of their rudder. And because girls with Turner Syndrome are slow to mature, it will take time and patience to help them take charge of their rudder.

Dealing with people and relationships can be challenging because of our social and behavioral deficits, and these are still challenging for me. Early on, it's important for the girl with NLD to be taught about the basic kinds of relationships, what appropriate boundaries are, and what is appropriate behavior within the various kinds of relationships. Behavior that might be appropriate within a family may not be appropriate with friends or coworkers. This is probably not going to be obvious for girls with NLD, so they must be taught and guided about it.

Social interactions can also be impacted by the fact that those with nonverbal learning disorder can also have problems with what is called "executive function." That is a set of mental skills that help you get things done, and it is controlled by the area of the brain called the frontal lobe. Among other things, the executive function helps you manage time, pay attention, switch focus, plan, and organize. Those with executive function issues have challenges both in school and out in the world because of the way our brains process information.

In essence, our ability to perceive and react, process and understand, store and retrieve information, make decisions, and produce appropriate results are all impacted by our problems with executive function. This is particularly relevant in our ability to face and deal with social situations and includes challenges with our ability to have relationships and understand basic interactions with others. This is why we have to be careful about who we surround ourselves with. Because we lack basic filters and understanding of our actions, we can be easily led. That can have catastrophic consequences, including being led into compromising actions and situations.

Miscommunication can also be a problem. There are times when I misinterpret what someone is saying to me. Because of that, if I think there may be a risk for miscommunication, I repeat my understanding of what the other person has said so they can clarify if I have misunderstood. Likewise, because of the way I present something, the person I'm talking to may not understand my meaning correctly. For this, I use many clues including body language, facial expression, and tone of voice. It helps if I'm face-to-face with the person I'm talking with or at least seeing them through a web conferencing platform. Unfortunately, many girls and women with TS have trouble looking directly at a person. This is not a nonverbal learning disorder issue, but because it *is* a Turner Syndrome issue, many women and girls who have both TS and NLD (the majority) will not have my ability to discern body language cues by looking at facial expression.

Among the issues related to rudder control for a Turner Syndrome girl with nonverbal learning disorder are anxiety and literal thinking. Without rudder control, the mind of a TS girl with nonverbal learning disorder may go to the worst-case scenario in any given situation. That is a part of her anxiety issues. And because she is likely to think in very literal terms, nuance can be lost on her.

Our literal thinking also affects something as simple as crossing the street. When there is a red light, I won't cross the street, even if there are no cars coming. I wait for the man walking sign. I won't go against the red light. Think about it: If you're driving your car and stop at a red light, even if there are no other cars around, you don't tell yourself that there are no cars coming, so you can run the red light. For those who think literally, the same rule applies to walking across the street. You don't cross when there is a red light.

One humorous note from my childhood regarding literal thinking is that I didn't understand sales tax when I purchased something. If I went to the store and the sticker on the item said $2.99, then that was what I paid. If I gave the cashier $3.00, I expected a penny back. I had no concept of sales tax and why they charged it. The family member with me generally had to make up the difference.

Because we are literal, those of us with nonverbal learning disorder are usually helped by setting up routines and giving us very specific instructions. That even applies to something as simple as getting dressed, which can be overwhelming for us. I like things done a certain way: I wash certain clothes together, fold cloths a certain way, and even wear certain things at certain times—right down to the accessories I wear with my clothes.

When you tell a NLD girl what to do and how to do it, that activity will become their routine. So where dressing is concerned, tell her the order in which to put on her clothes and give her the same order to put them on the next time you instruct her how to get dressed (which you will have to do because of our need for repetition—the lather, rinse, repeat requirement). If you tell her to put on her underwear, then her shirt, then her socks one time and tell her to put on her underwear, socks, and shirt the next time, you will likely confuse her. And when she's confused, she may have a meltdown.

Some girls with Turner Syndrome and NLD will, like me, be able to handle change if you gently show us the way. For me, that includes showing me how the change will work and what the end result will be.

Earlier I mentioned being able to give speeches at Toastmasters but having trouble with table topics because impromptu speaking is not one of my strong suits. Literal thinking is one reason for that. During table topics, you have to speak spontaneously and concisely in response to a topic you are given without prior preparation. But not only does the information required to respond need to already be in my memory banks, I need time to think about and organize my answer because I'm being taken out of my routine way of thinking and responding.

The impact of executive function difficulties for those with NLD affects us throughout our lives. It impacts our ability in school when abstract thinking is involved and in our lives both in and out of school with things like time management and organizing both things and ideas. We may struggle to apply learning in one area to others and may compartmentalize, which creates difficulty with integrating ideas or concepts into a coherent whole. Because routine is helpful to us, when we need to do something new, like drive to an unfamiliar location or take an alternative route to get somewhere, we may struggle. And our difficulties with time management, organization, and social interactions can impact our job performance.

Because the impact of nonverbal learning disorder is so pervasive, it is important to understand this condition early in your daughter's life and learn how to work with your daughter on it if she has it.

- **Lesson 1:** *Many girls with Turner Syndrome also have nonverbal learning disorder (NLD). How it impacts her can vary.*

- **Lesson 2:** *NLD impacts many aspects of a Turner Syndrome girl's life, so it is important to identify it and learn how to help her manage it.*

- **Lesson 3:** *With NLD, your daughter will not understand that she has an internal rudder, let alone how to use it, until you teach her these things and work with her on them.*

- **Lesson 4:** *Turner Syndrome girls with NLD will probably like routines, have difficulty with change, and take things literally.*

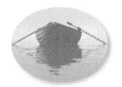

CHAPTER 3

Rudders and Relationships

BECAUSE OF THE WAY OR BRAIN WORKS, those of us with Turner Syndrome are often clueless about a lot of things. As mentioned earlier, one way of describing it for the majority of TS girls who also have nonverbal learning disorder is to say that our brain is adrift in a boat without a rudder. And without a rudder, it's easy for us to get into to trouble because external forces drive us.

Let's say someone with TS is in a store with a friend who sees something she would like to have and says, "Just put this lipstick in your purse for me." The girl with Turner Syndrome may do exactly what they are asked. And because her friend is in charge of her rudder at that moment, the girl with TS doesn't openly question what she is being asked to do. That's why we have to be careful about who are friends and acquaintances are.

Those of us with TS mature a little slowly, but we get there. We need what are considered to be normal parameters of behavior explained to us because we are rudderless, adrift on the river of life, and otherwise won't know the rules. Since we are behind in maturity, we may not be able to ascertain what is socially acceptable behavior and what is not. For instance, we may open the front door to an unknown adult and let them enter the house. Obviously, that could lead to any number of catastrophic consequences: They might take what does not belong to them or lead us into questionable behavior because we don't have the internal discernment needed to know better.

One way this lack of maturity and discernment impacts me, personally, is that when I mention I want to do something with another person, I want and expect to be able to do it immediately. And if it cannot take place immediately, I want to be told when it will happen. For instance, if I suggest going to a movie with a friend, I may either want my friend to go to the movie with me that day or tell me which day they can go to the movie with me. If I'm given a vague answer like, "Yes, let's go to a movie sometime," I may feel ignored and insignificant in their life.

This personal idiosyncrasy is not only a matter of immaturity and lack of discernment, it also relates to other challenges that TS and NLD girls have: challenges with perception—how we perceive things and how we present things to others. With nonverbal learning disorder, you feel you are on the outside looking in. For example, when I'm in a social or work situation with more than one other person and feel excluded, I have to ask myself if they are deliberately leaving me out or if it is just my impression colored by my NLD.

If you are the parent of a daughter with Turner Syndrome and the NLD that often accompanies it, assure your daughter that while she *is* different and may *feel* she is on the outside looking in, you can help her manage her perceptions. Show her how to take a mental break and evaluate what is going on. Help her to examine whether her perception is accurate or is actually colored by her NLD.

It is also helpful to discuss relationships in general. Family relationships are different from relationships with friends, neighbors, classmates, and others. So are the expectations associated with each type of relationship. Talking with her about this will help her avoid having unrealistic expectations of herself and others. Every type of relationship has a different level of personal investment, and when the investments on both ends are in sync, you have the best possible chance for a healthy relationship. By helping her understand how different kinds of relationships are formed and sustained, you will be helping your daughter navigate her relationships with fewer misunderstandings and more ease.

Here is an example of what a conversation might look like.

Lisa, an eight-year-old girl with Turner Syndrome, is playing in the park with three friends. Her father is nearby. Suddenly she runs up to her father crying. He enfolds her in his arms and asks, "What's the matter?"

She sobs, "They don't like me."

Lisa has Turner Syndrome and non-verbal learning disorder, so he knows he needs to ask some questions to fully understand the situation. "You mean Michelle, Tammy, and Debbie?"

She nods her head against his shoulder.

He pulls a bit away from her to wipe her tears. "What makes you think they don't like you?"

Unable to articulate why she feels her friends don't like her, she just shrugs.

"Okay, close your eyes for a moment," her says. "Picture yourself and the girls playing. What were you doing?"

"We were swinging."

"Good. What else happened?"

"They were talking."

"And?"

"They weren't talking to me," Lisa replies through her sobs.

"I know you love to talk. Did you try talking to them?"

Lisa lowers her head. "No."

"Okay. Did you try to say something and they told you to shut up?"

"No."

"Did you try to say something and they ignored you, continuing to talk and pretending you hadn't said anything?"

"No"

"Good. Open your eyes now."

Lisa looks into her father's eyes.

"If any of those things had happened, then I would say you're right," he says. "But none of those things happened. Because you think differently than they do, you can feel left out, like they don't like you. It sounds like they were taking turns talking and you didn't take your turn.

"Try to think about how you can take a turn next time. And when you feel you're being left out, do what we just did. Think about what just happened. If you realize you haven't been joining in on the conversation, think about how you can take your turn talking. And if you feel you're being deliberately ignored, tell them how that makes you feel. Don't just get upset and start crying.

"Nothing is going to change if you stay quiet or cry and get upset. Also, because they think differently than you, they may not know you're feeling left out. Your feelings are your feelings, and that's okay. You just need to learn what to do with them."

Those kinds of conversations will help your daughter in many social situations. But some social situations require a bit more planning and thought. You will need to search your morals, values, and religious beliefs before you have "the talk" with your daughter, but you *will* need to have a talk with her. Fortunately, some things are applicable in any relationship, not just those involving romance. How does he (or she) treat your daughter when they are around friends and family? If he does not consistently treat your daughter with respect, he is not worthy of her time.

I never had any kind of a talk with my mom, and I was immature for my age, so when members of the opposite sex started showing interest in me, I didn't understand how to respond. Consequently, I missed out on having romantic relationships.

Relationships are not only a normal part of life, they are critical to managing our lives successfully. Your TS daughter will need gentle, consistent guidance from you to learn how to behave appropriately and manage relationships of all kinds.

• **Lesson:** *Because girls with TS and NLD are rudderless, they may have trouble understanding how to behave appropriately in social situations. Talk to your daughter about socially acceptable behavior, perceptions, relationships, and respect.*

CHAPTER 4

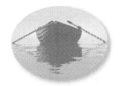

Negative Self-Talk

THOSE WITH TURNER SYNDROME have a super power: our memory. Our brain records everything we see and hear. It is as if we have a recording device within us that picks up and records everything. Because of this ability, we have superior recall and retention. We can replay what we have "recorded" in a way that is very much like watching a video or listening to an audio recording. And it does not matter how long ago we "recorded" what we saw or heard. It could have been five minutes ago or fifty years ago.

Growing up, my brother—just being a typical big brother—told me I was stupid and would never amount to anything. Realistically, he probably only said it once or twice, but because he was older than me, because he was family, and because I saw him as an authority figure, I thought it must be true. One of my sisters told me I was selfish and ungrateful. That was also recorded in my memory banks. All that negative input became my mantra, and the recording telling me I was stupid, selfish, and ungrateful and that I wouldn't amount to anything ran in my head continually for most of my life.

I read—and still read—a lot of books. Though mostly I read for enjoyment, sometimes I read to drown out or still the recording playing in my head that repeats what my brother said to me. At some level, I believe that if I read enough books, own them, and gain enough knowledge from them, I won't be dumb. No matter what you read, you can always learn something if you pay attention.

It wasn't until I reached my fifties and started listening to Stephen Covey, Zig Ziglar, Norman Vincent Peal, and Brian Tracy that I began learning about changing the channel I was playing in my head and how to switch those negative mental recordings.

We dwell on our negative self-talk, and by doing that, we are constantly waiting for the other shoe to drop. We continually come up with negative outcomes that haven't yet happened. And even if something *has* happened, it's usually not as bad as we imagined it could be. That's probably why I left some of the jobs I've had over the years: I didn't want to wait and see what else they would throw at me.

An example of waiting for the other shoe to drop happened when I wanted my house remodeled. The impetus to begin the project was that my new dishwasher leaked water and had destroyed my kitchen floor. The company I hired took up the floor and subflooring and promised to put plywood down before they left for the day. Because they were also remodeling my bathroom and it was torn up, I had no bathroom sink at the moment. If they put plywood down, I would at least have access to the kitchen sink, and I wouldn't be concerned about my cats falling into the crawl space.

But they did not do this. I had gaping holes in my floor for almost twelve hours. It was too dangerous for me to get to the kitchen sink, and the only way to keep my cats out of the kitchen was to isolate them in my home office until the contractors left the next day. This meant my cats were in my office for slightly more than twenty-four hours.

I cried myself to sleep thinking my house was going to be condemned and I would be forced to live on the street. Overly dramatic? Yes. I came up with the worst-case scenario. It wasn't just a matter of a problem I had to deal with for one night. I imagined that utter tragedy would result, and I had a terrible night as I waited for the other shoe to drop.

Another example of what a Turner Syndrome brain can do in a situation is the second-guessing that happens sometimes when I receive gifts. For instance, when I have been given perfume or bath sets as presents in the past, my immediate reaction has been to wonder if I'm being told that I smell or need a bath. I have to take a step back, think, and reframe the situation: *These are normal, standard gifts. You're reading too much into it.*

A more recent example is when my brother had his gallbladder removed. It was to be an outpatient procedure, and the hospital's requirement was that someone be at the hospital during the operation. My brother's ex-wife was supposed to take him to the hospital, stay with him, and then take him home. Unfortunately, she reneged, sending everyone into a slight panic trying to find someone who was in a position to help.

I was eventually asked to step in, but it seemed that I was an afterthought because they talked about others who might be able to help before I was asked. My feelings were also colored by my NLD perceptions. It felt like they weren't sure I would be willing to do it or that if I *was* willing, I wouldn't have the mental capacity to help. But of course I was willing. He is, after all, my brother.

Once we were back at his house after the procedure, I was asked how he was doing and given suggestions by text on how to take care of him—which made me feel they were questioning my competence. When my sister finally said it sounded like I had everything under control, I asked her if she'd thought I *wouldn't* have had it under control and if she would have handled things differently. She replied, "Nope." That one word made me feel good, and I realized she was just making suggestions because she wasn't there, didn't know what was happening, and wanted to be helpful. She wasn't actually questioning my abilities.

All of these examples point to the fact that a person with Turner Syndrome may interpret situations based on old misunderstandings and negative self-talk running in their brains. If you are the parent (friend, colleague, family member, boss) of someone with Turner Syndrome, it's helpful to ask them questions about what they're thinking and feeling, especially if you suspect they may be misinterpreting or catastrophizing a situation. Not only is it important for *you* to ask questions, it is important to let the person with Turner Syndrome know that it's okay for *her* to ask questions of her family, trusted friends, counselor, and boss.

Because those of us with TS and NLD lack a sense of direction, it is easy for us to float down the river, rudderless, and just let things happen instead of making things happen. And while we're floating down that river, we're probably running old stories and beliefs in our head.

It goes back to an old computer programming adage: garbage in, garbage out. What you put into your mind affects your perceptions and impacts what you put out. If you ever want to know what we're thinking, just ask. We're auditory and love to talk. We'd be happy to tell you what we are mentally telling ourselves. If you are a parent of someone with TS, you can use that information to help your daughter craft new mental self-talk. You can also help her create strategies for catching herself lapsing into old patterns of negative self-talk and switch to those new, healthier internal messages.

• **Lesson:** *Those of us with Turner Syndrome tend to dwell on the conclusions we've come to that may be the result of misunderstandings or negative self-talk. That is why it is so important for us to learn to ask questions of others and for those in our lives to ask us questions. By asking questions, we can discover if what we are*

mentally telling ourselves about what we are experiencing is correct or incorrect. And when we challenge our limiting beliefs, we are freed up to ask even more questions that may help us discover and pursue our passions, seek out opportunities, and turn possibilities into realities instead of just continuing to float down the river. When those in our lives ask us questions, they can determine what we are telling ourselves that does not serve us and help change it if needed.

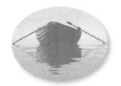

CHAPTER 5

Respect and Being Different

WHAT I REMEMBER MOST about growing up is watching TV. Anytime I tried to do anything else or join in discussions held in the kitchen, I was told to go watch TV. If I tried to say anything about what I needed or wanted, I was told I was being selfish or ungrateful. I also remember being told, "No one wants to hear it, Mary." Can you imagine telling that to someone with TS who deals strictly with the auditory form of communication? Realistically, I was probably only told those things a handful of times, but because those speaking were members of my family—my authority figures, my elders—I let them control my rudder. What they said went onto my mental tapes and became part of what consistently played in my head.

Needless to say, I became absorbed in TV. In fact, at one time, I wanted to be an actress, and I became fixated on it because I wanted to be someone else. People with nonverbal learning disorder typically want to be someone else because they think they would be liked and/or loved if they were someone else.

I certainly felt that way growing up. I felt set aside and ignored as a child. As the youngest of six children, with some of my siblings significantly older than me, birth order might explain a part of how I felt. My older siblings, particularly those who were teenagers, had their own friends and activities and likely were not interested in spending time with a small child. But at least some of those feelings could be attributed to my TS and NLD perception. Because of my small size and my cognitive differences, I got verbally and physically patted on the head (even when I wasn't being tortured by my older brother). And in fact, there have been instances throughout my life when, because of my small stature, I've felt treated with less respect than I deserved.

But being different doesn't have to lead to feelings of being disrespected, set aside, and ignored. You can help your daughter see that being different can not only be okay, it can be good. Let me give you a hypothetical example.

Katlyn, a twelve-year-old girl with Turner Syndrome, complains to her parents about being short and dumb. "I hate it, just hate it! I hate being short! And I'm so stupid, I can't do math or English!

"You're cute like a pixie," her father replies, "and some people happen to prefer pixies."

She rolls her eyes, and with a flourish of hand movements says, "Women don't want to be pixies. They want to be beautiful and glamorous."

"Hmm," her father says. "So you're saying Eva Longoria, Jada Pinkett Smith, and Dolly Pardon aren't beautiful and glamorous? What about Mary Lou Retton? And remember *The Wizard of Oz*? Judy Garland played Dorothy in that. How about her? And what about Ruth Bader-Ginsberg? Wasn't she a knockout in court? They're all short women. In fact, Mary Lou Retton is four-foot-nine. And even the tallest of them is only a little more than five feet. It's all in how you carry yourself, think about yourself, and dress the package. We can help you work on those things."

The wheels began turning in Katlyn's head. "RBG? Eva? Really? You think I can be smart like Ruth? What about being beautiful like Eva?

"You can do whatever you want to do. If you want to be glamourous like Eva, you can learn how to do that. We can help you. If you want to be a trailblazer like Ruth, we can help with that too."

"But I can't write and I can barely put two plus two together to make four."

Katlyn's mom put her arm around her daughter's shoulder. "You can do it. It will just take a little more work because your brain processes information differently than others. Think about it this way: Someone with dyslexia isn't dumb. They just process information differently. They can be taught and they can learn. So can you. We'll ask your teachers for help in figuring this out."

As the parent of a girl with TS and NLD, you can help your daughter reframe being "different" and help her see that being different is not only okay, it can be a good thing.

• **Lesson 1:** *Treat the person in your life who has Turner Syndrome with respect. Don't pat her on the head and tell her it's okay when she doesn't understand something. Take the time to explain it to her. She does*

not have diminished capacities and is capable of under-standing. She just thinks differently, and it may take her a little time to get it.

- **Lesson 2:** *Help her understand what it means to be different and that being different is okay. Help her find her voice and be her biggest cheerleader.*

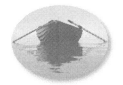

CHAPTER 6

The Hallowed Halls of Academia

PEOPLE WITH nonverbal learning disorder typically have challenges in school. Usually, those challenges include things like difficulty focusing and multitasking, problems with reading comprehension and essay writing, and trouble with math skills.

I only had a few challenges. The first was flunking second grade. My teacher never talked to me about flunking, and no one—including my mother—inquired about the reasons for it. When we moved to Colorado that summer, my mother had my sister try to reenroll me in second grade. Thank God for the principal, Mr. Spokstra. "Why don't we put her in third grade and see how she does?" he said to my sister. So I went into the third grade and did just fine.

I was lucky. I wasn't held back. When I was in elementary school, there was no understanding of Turner Syndrome or nonverbal learning disorder. Dr. Henry Turner first described what came to be known as Turner Syndrome in 1938, but it wasn't until 1960 that the chromosome connection was discovered. And nonverbal learning disorder was not discovered until about 1970. So while my challenges in school were probably related to TS and NLD, no one could have identified what was causing my problems at the time.

I managed my way through school okay until my second semester of geometry in high school. First semester was fine. The teacher let us write out the theorems so we could have cheat sheets for tests. But in second semester, I was switched to a different teacher, and we had to memorize the theorems. That required me to not only memorize the theorems introduced in second semester but memorize those from first semester as well. I couldn't do it. I gave up and got an F.

Neither my teacher nor my mother asked why my grade dropped so drastically, but neither could have made the connection to Turner Syndrome because it was only just beginning to be understood in the medical community at the time.

What we now know is that TS people tend to be auditory. We learn by listening. That doesn't work well with learning math, and in fact, most TS people have trouble with math. We generally need to be able to *hear* what we are being asked to memorize spoken, so it is no surprise that I had trouble memorizing Geometry theorems.

I also had challenges with English. Those of us with nonverbal learning disorder typically have problems putting down on paper what we're thinking, and because we may have trouble with fine motor skills, our handwriting can be atrocious. But we are often very creative. My high school English teacher couldn't comprehend why I couldn't understand such simple things as nouns, pronouns, conjunctions, or dangling participles. (To this day, I can't tell you the definition of any of them.) She went to my drama teacher and asked how I did memorizing lines. My drama teacher told her I could memorize lines just fine. Neither of them understood that I had nonverbal learning disorder, so they could not understand that the superpower for NLD people is memory. Because of that, drama was my strong suit, not English.

I continued to have problems with English in college. My English teacher took me aside and told me that I was going to flunk freshman English if I didn't change it from a graded class to an audited one. I met with my advisor and audited the class. The following semester, I took it as a graded class and earned a C, which I felt good about because it meant my work was satisfactory and I was meeting standards.

If you're the parent of a Turner Syndrome daughter with nonverbal learning disorder, you can help her have an easier time than I had because both individual education programs (IEPs) and special education classes are often available. IEPs can work if two things happen. First, the child needs to be directly involved in the decision-making process. They know what works for them and what motivates them.

They may not be able to describe how they learn best (such as by listening or by reading), so you need to listen to how they describe their environment. For example, how I would describe my school days is that all I had to do was go to class to get a C or a B in that subject. If I cracked a book, I would get an A or a B. In other words, if I just went to class and listened to the teacher, I would get a C or even a B, but if I also read the material, I would often get an A. This would clue anyone in who is paying attention that my favorite mode of learning is auditory but that I also have high comprehension with reading.

Of course, the combination of hearing problems, which most TS girls have, and our tendency to be auditory explains a part of why I always sat at the front of the class. But there was more to it than that. It was also related to the fact that I was short and needed glasses to see the chalkboard.

It is essential that the parent and teacher cooperate with one another and with the TS/NLD girl. Sometimes there is a battle of wills with the parent and the teacher each thinking they know what is best for the child. Both need to put their egos aside and listen to what the child says she needs.

Special education classes are another option, but you need to evaluate several criteria. First, observe and talk with the teacher. Some more naturally fit the needs of this group than others. Next, look at the culture of the school. How are people who are "different" treated? Children have a tendency to think they would be liked if they were someone other than who they are: taller, thinner, prettier, smarter, more athletic, funnier—whatever. As stated earlier, those with NLD often want to be someone else. You need to help them accept themselves for who they are, and that includes paying attention to the messages they are getting about themselves from teachers and schoolmates.

- **Lesson:** *You can only meet your daughter's educational needs when you listen to her and understand how she learns best and what she needs. When you truly listen, you can work on developing a game plan that works for her. Additionally, if you are involved in her education and work with her to understand her world, being clear that you can only help her if she lets you know what she needs will teach her to ask for what she needs when she starts college and enters the workforce.*

CHAPTER 7

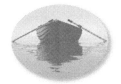

Put Up Your Dukes

ALONG WITH THE educational aspects of school, you need to have a discussion with your daughter about bullying because school is where bullying often starts. Find out how her school handles bullying, and help your child learn that it is not okay to be bullied and that they have permission to speak up should bullying occur. Help them develop a game plan if they are bullied.

Turner Syndrome girls may be more prone to bullying than other girls because they are short and because they often present as naïve and innocent—almost to the point of appearing gullible. That was certainly the case with me.

A couple of classmates—cousins to one another—thought they could pick on me. One day after school, I noticed that they were following me and whispering to one another. It didn't feel right to me, so I decided to go home a different way than I usually did. But they were still following me, so I circled back around and tried hiding behind the school stairs. Unfortunately, that didn't work. They found me, said ugly things, and slapped me around. A couple of girls walked by, saw what was happening, and asked why they were doing that to me. With clenched fists at her side, one of the bullies took a step towards them and said, "Because we can." Intimidated, the girls moved on.

I finally made it home, and my mother must have been able to see that something serious had transpired because she asked me what had happened. I tried to brush it off because the bullying cousins said they would get me worse if I said anything, but I finally told her about the bullying. The next day, my teacher asked me and the two bullies to stay after school. She pointedly looked at the cousins and said,

"You know why you're here." Then she turned to me and told me I could go. Whatever she said or did to them, that form of bullying stopped for the rest of that year.

The same bullies came after me another time—and with a worse outcome for me. It had just snowed, and a couple of other kids and I were making a snowman. I had just gotten a new skirt that looked like a Scottish tartan. It was the first and only time I wore that skirt. As we were finishing our snowman, the cousins pushed me into the chain-link fence, which chipped a front tooth and cut my lips. As I cried, blood got on everything, and it totally ruined my new skirt. They grabbed my arms and took me to the school nurse, all the while saying, "Don't cry. It's not that bad."

My mom took me in for emergency dental work. The dentist filed down my tooth and told my mom to bring me back when I was fourteen to put a cap on it. I never went back, and the tooth was never capped.

The bullying continued in junior high. In the lunch line one day, a boy was trash talking about me to his friends, who were eating it up and laughing. What he failed to notice was that I kept getting closer and closer to him. Finally, when I got close enough, I was so boiling mad that I kicked him in the shin. His friends laughed and embarrassed him because a girl—and a short one at that—had gotten the best of him. I'm not advocating violence in response to bullying, but he never bothered me again.

Another time in junior high, a girl and her friends came up to me and asked to see my purse. Always the innocent, I handed it over to the girl. It wasn't until later that I realized my lunch money was missing. She had taken it. I went to the school office and talked to the vice-principle. I never knew what he did about it, but she never bothered me again._

In high school, things were a little different. I carried a big bag . . . with lots of stuff in it. Get the picture? If anyone said anything derogatory within my hearing, I just gave my *big* bag a swing. The *Family Matters* character, Urquelle, used to say, "Did I do that?" I had that perfected before he was a glimmer in anyone's eye. People learned to avoid saying anything demeaning about me within my earshot because I wasn't going to take *anything* from anyone.

I have no doubt that I didn't handle the instances of bullying very well, but I played the cards I was dealt and had little help when it came to creating appropriate tactics to manage bullying. That is why you must discuss this topic with your daughters and develop a more appropriate way of dealing with bullying.

I discovered a new way to look at bullying during a sermon my pastor gave one Christmas. He started with Matthew 5:39-41—the passage that talks about turning the other cheek, handing over both your cloak and shirt if someone sues you for your cloak, and going two miles if a man forces you to go one. While this may sound as if Christians are supposed to be milquetoast and a rug on which others can wipe their feet, nothing could be further from the truth. What the passage is trying to do is show people how ridiculous and stupid bullying is.

You see, the custom at the time was to backhand an individual to humiliate them and put them in their place. That would be done with the right hand, landing the blow on the individual's left cheek. So if the person being hit turned the other cheek, the bully would have to backhand them again, but this time, using their left hand. And using the left hand was unacceptable. According to Semitic society at that time, the left hand was unclean and used only for unclean tasks.

According to my pastor's sermon, striking someone with the back of the hand was meant to put someone in their place, not physically hurt them. So Jesus's advice was that if someone tried to humiliate you and put you in an inferior position, you should turn the other cheek, which would force them to recognize they were doing something unclean. It also shows how stupid bullying is because backhanding someone twice is like telling a joke twice. If they didn't get it the first time, its purpose had failed. By turning the other cheek, you stand defiantly saying, "I refuse to be humiliated by you." And in doing so, you keep your dignity.

What about giving someone your shirt, as well as your cloak, if you're sued for your cloak? They're a bully if they take your cloak, but if the person who has sued you for the cloak is willing to also take your shirt, it reveals to everyone just how big a bully they are. And how about going two miles when forced to go one? This relates to the fact that Roman soldiers were allowed to force Jews to carry their backpacks for a mile. By going two miles instead of one, the person being pressed into service is showing their ability to rise above the bullying.

Help your daughters stand up to bullies triumphantly and defiantly. Let them know that they should not allow themselves to be humiliated. Help them find ways to understand that bullying is a black mark on the bully, not on their target, and it is both pointless and stupid.

• **Lesson:** *Bullying is not acceptable! Research how your daughter's school handles bullying, and talk to your daughter about bullying and how to deal with it. Support your daughter in accepting herself and her differences and teach her to stand up for herself, when needed, in healthy, nonviolent ways.*

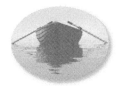

CHAPTER 8

Entering the Workforce

DISCOVERING HER STRENGTHS and weaknesses will help your daughter decide on a career for herself and thrive in that career, and you can assist her in that discovery process. Notice that I didn't say *job*. Jobs have limits. But a career can evolve as you change and grow. A career is something you feel so passionately about that you're willing to devote a big chunk of your life to it.

There are a few challenges to consider when entering the workforce. The first challenge is that those of us with Turner Syndrome are very literal. I see things in black-and-white. I'm aware that shades of grey exist. I just need to help see those options.

Another challenge that your daughter may have is communication problems related to her hearing and the way her brain works. I have learned to repeat my understanding of a task back to the person giving it to me and any instructions related to it.

But even weaknesses can often be turned into strengths. For instance, I turned my ability to think literally into an asset. I used it to help my boss craft clearer and more easily understood communications, policies, and procedures. I'm also able to see small details, and one of my bosses joked that I not only saw the trees in the forest, I saw the woodpecker three trees over and four trees back. She realized this could be an asset to her, and it was my job to let her know if that woodpecker was going to affect the forest.

I never used my college degree in theater because my family couldn't figure out what I could do with it, and I never talked to my college advisor about it. I didn't know I could seek guidance from her or how valuable that guidance might be, nor did I know she could help me find a career in which I could use my degree. And without guidance, I had no real idea about how to create a plan for my future. Using the floating down the river metaphor, my family was in charge of the rudder of my boat, and I was not allowed to pursue acting. Actually, in this case, a car metaphor might be more accurate because I was in a car with my brother and mother when I announced that I wanted to be an actress. My brother stopped the car. He and my mother, who was in the front passenger seat, turned to look at me in the back seat and laughed.

Wanting to be an actress wasn't just an idle fantasy. Over the years since that announcement, I've taken acting workshops, and a couple of workshop teachers who actually worked in the field said I would have made a terrific character actress. I would definitely not have been the first actress with Turner Syndrome. Award-winning actress Linda Hunt has Turner Syndrome, and that didn't prevent her from winning an Oscar. I wanted to go to New York to see if I could get a job in theater, but since I couldn't tell my family exactly what type of a job I would look for, I was told that wasn't an option.

If I'd had some help discovering and exploring my strengths and weaknesses, I might have been clearer about how I could make a career for myself in the theatrical arts. This is where working with a guidance counselor would have been beneficial.

My mother suggested I get a degree in computer science, and because she was in charge of my otherwise rudderless boat, I listened to her, even though I wasn't interested in computer science. As it turned out, I was good at it. And while I did get a degree in that field, I never got a job using that degree for several reasons. One reason was that I observed my job applications being thrown in the trash by secretaries more than once. I felt it was because I looked so young, but whatever the reason, my applications sometimes didn't even get to the hiring manager.

Another reason I didn't work in that field was that my mother and brother debated in front of me whether I even had enough intelligence to get a job flipping burgers at McDonalds. They were probably talking about social intelligence and social skills, not brain power, because I'd already demonstrated that I had the mental horsepower to complete two degrees. But because I, like other TS girls, took things literally, I believed they didn't think I had enough intelligence to flip burgers. I quit pursuing jobs because I didn't believe I could convince an employer I was intelligent enough to be hired if my own family didn't think I was.

But a third reason really cinched it. When I found out my mother was dying, I believed there was no time to pursue jobs and put in applications. I needed to take the first job I could find. Living life without a rudder and just floating down the river landed me a minimum wage job a Chuck E. Cheese.

There are several incidents while working at Chuck E. Cheese that are worth reflecting on. While working there, one of the managers prepared a written reprimand on me without cause. She accused me of failing to do something that had never actually been a part of my job. I didn't realize I could question the writeup, so I didn't. Fortunately, I had the support of another manager, so it did little harm, but if I had known I could stand up for myself and the appropriate way to do that, I would have been better off.

I also got written up the first time I cashiered because my drawer came up seven dollars short. After that writeup, the manager on duty taught me a trick to help me keep track of what was going out of my drawer and what was coming in using the images on the bills and whether they were facing right or left. And because I was a literal thinker, that worked for me. I obsessively made sure the bills faced the right way for receiving money and for handing it out. I loved it, and I was never more than a few cents off after that. In fact, I amused my favorite manager one time when he told me my drawer was a penny off and I handed him a penny I'd found earlier that day on the floor saying, "Oh, you mean this penny?" He cracked up laughing. Sometimes what is considered a challenge can be turned into an advantage.

The third incident reflects something more concerning, and it is something all Turner Syndrome girls and women have to watch out for. An individual from the corporate office came to interview all staff. I had heard a couple of individuals talking about how bad a particular manager was, and when it was my turn to talk to the corporate official, I repeated what I'd overheard about the manager, even though it was not my personal experience. Coworkers had said it was true, so I thought it must be true. I wasn't in control of my own rudder, and I'd taken what others had said literally. It was a mistake for me to repeat what I'd heard, and I did that manager a disservice by it.

When Chuck E. Cheese went bankrupt, I got a job as a part-time receptionist at a furniture manufacturing company. I answered the phones, tracked inventory, and processed orders. It was an easy job, and I liked it. But I needed full-time work, so I eventually took a full-time job as a receptionist at another company. When the office manager there left, I took on some of her duties. I impressed the corporate office because my computer background helped me clear up a computer glitch that was interfering with the transmission of daily reports.

Unfortunately, that didn't help me when a new boss took over. Whatever his expectations were, I apparently didn't meet them, and I was fired. What I didn't understand was that I should have initiated a conversation with him about his expectations when he took over. I was continuing to just float down the river.

I had rent and student loans to pay, so I thought about what I could do. I went to work for a temp agency, and they placed me in a bookkeeping job at a hospital's senior clinic. I took care of their Medicare log. I was so good at it, the hospital hired me on, and I became an asset to them because of my ability to think literally and pay attention to small details. When I was a penny off in my books one year, my manager told me it would be okay to fudge it. My literal mind wouldn't let me do it, and like a bloodhound, I went in search of that missing penny. I discovered it was masking a six-cent error. It was a small thing, but the same mind that unearthed small errors had the ability to keep larger errors from happening.

After I left the senior clinic, I ran into a college friend who was the leasing coordinator for a low-income housing organization run by nuns, and she suggested I get a job there. The housing complex had a section for seniors and a section for families, and when I got a job with them, I began as a receptionist in the senior area and then worked as a leasing agent for the entire complex.

I had both challenges and triumphs working for the low-income housing organization. In the challenges department was the bus. I needed to take a bus to get to my job, and it took me a while before I got the hang of catching the bus that would actually get me to my work on time. Before I resolved that problem, I was late enough times that it almost cost me my job. As for triumphs, one of them happened during a medical emergency in which I managed to keep everyone calm, including the person in crisis, until the paramedics arrived. And it did not go unnoticed. I was deemed good in a crisis by my leasing coordinator friend.

I had to make thoughtful decisions in that position, and those of us with Turner Syndrome really have challenges with decisions, especially if they affect other people. A coworker and I met to interview a wonderful woman applying for the senior portion of the complex. Unfortunately, a fire had destroyed the files where she had been living and the manager there had died, so there wasn't ten years of information available. The board had stipulated that they needed ten years' worth of information in a previous meeting, and I took that literally. I was insistent during the interview that we had to have a full ten years of information. The poor woman became upset and withdrew her application. The board might have made an exception in her case, but I was focused on the rule that we needed ten years of information, and I was determined to get it. We lost what would have likely been a good resident because of it.

Having to make decisions was scary, but I liked the fact this low-income housing organization used theatrical productions as one way to bring together those in the senior section with the families in the non-senior part of the housing complex. The groups had a tendency to be at odds with each other, so the organization used this as a way of bringing them together in a noncombative way. I loved this because I got to perform in the productions. In *A Christmas*

Carol, I was both Scrooge's fiancé and the Ghost of Christmas Past. And in *The King and I*, I was given the role of Anna. I was also Annie in the play *Annie*. I loved the costumes, I loved performing—I just loved all of it.

When I eventually left that organization and went back to work at a temp agency, I was placed in a mailroom position at a big corporation. In that position, I discovered another skill, but it had nothing to do with sorting mail. We had a mentally handicapped young girl working with us. She had taken ill and had been out of the mailroom for about a week. When she returned, I saw her with another woman in the hallway. The woman was trying to talk to her, and she kept shaking her head no, acting like she was nervous. I was able to empathize with the young girl. I thought about how I would feel being gone from work for a week. I had been watching the interaction through a window, and I went into the hall, took her by the hand, and said I was glad to see her because we had been waiting for her to come back. Then I took her to her desk and showed her that nothing had changed. She still had her own desk and her own items to work with. She smiled and immediately got to work.

Later, one of the leads told me that the woman who had been trying to talk with her in the hallway was her social worker and the social worker said I had done exactly the right thing to help my coworker. That made me feel really good. Perhaps my challenges with Turner Syndrome, nonverbal learning disorder, and life in general had helped teach me how to empathize with others. In any event, it was fulfilling to know I had helped my coworker and had been recognized by both the social worker and lead worker for it.

But again, I needed something permanent, not temporary. I found work as a receptionist for a retirement community with an assisted living section. I eventually became their activities director, and I liked the work but never liked the wording in the job description because it sounded as if I alone was responsible for the residents participating in activities. That concerned me because I felt that if something happened to a resident, I was on my own with no backup from the organization. I didn't understand that I could ask for the wording in the contract to be clarified before I signed it. I just felt the corporation was not going to stand by me should something happen, and rather than going to bat for myself, I started looking for another job.

My brother had been after me to get a job with the City and County of Denver. Eventually, after multiple rounds of testing, I did get a job with the city working in the department that was going to be responsible for redeveloping the old airport site. Later, the city decided that a private corporation should redevelop the site, and I was sent out to the new airport to work. I was basically a receptionist in the "properties" office, but I ended up doing much more than that classification, and an audit on my position was requested. That led to a promotion.

Because of my determination and work ethic, I became known as the pit bull of the airport. I knew so much about everything that I had the call center employees calling me for advice on who could help

whom. Things went well, and I had great performance evaluations. I had multiple people giving me
things to do in my work role, and I learned to ask,
"When do you need this by?" That helped me prior-
itize my work.

I had one hiccup. One of the managers I sup-
ported asked me to mail something for him. He
handed me a packet that contained financial information for several people and said, "Mail this" instead
of "Mail these." With my literal mind, I sent the
whole thing to one person. It was a big mistake. The
person receiving the packet notified his lawyer. His
lawyer called my boss and asked him why his client
had gotten financial records for several other people.
My boss was very angry, and when he asked me how
that had happened, I had a hard time explaining that
I had taken what the manager said literally. Remember, those with TS are seldom good at extemporaneous speaking. I just couldn't get that thought out.
Fortunately, I had a good track record in that position,
so I didn't lose my job. But I began wondering what
more there might be out there for me.

I discovered that a secretarial position at the city's television station was available. I thought it would be a good extension of my liberal arts/theater background, so I applied and got the job. I was only there for a couple of months because the person I reported to would not explain what she wanted done and how she wanted it done. She just wouldn't talk to me, and how could I do my job if she wouldn't talk to an auditory person like me? And I need direction or I will just float on down the river. But asking this individual questions was not an option. I eventually went back to the airport.

The department I was assigned to at the airport was the customer service department. The largest portion of my time was spent crunching numbers concerning questions the customer service agents were asked, and a part of my time was spent working on sick leave slips. Among other things, the sick leave slips were used for overtime calculations. I talked to the payroll department about the correct way to calculate them and used that method, but the supervisors wanted them calculated a different way.

That caused a problem, and the supervisors went to the manager over the issue.

When it came time for my performance review, the manager put in my evaluation that I was a danger to the people in my department. What he meant was that he thought I was a danger to the authority of the supervisors because I had sided with payroll over the supervisors on the overtime calculation issue. I read the statement several times, and my literal mind definitely read it as a statement that I was a physical danger to the department supervisors. And I felt others would read it that way too. I was concerned enough to go to human resources with the issue. They agreed with me. I grieved the review wording, and the wording was changed. For once, I had stood up for myself, and the issue was taken seriously.

Eventually, I was transferred to the airport volunteer program, and over the next several years, I had both good and bad experiences. One goodhearted manager wouldn't let me do much, which didn't work well for me because I didn't have enough to do. Because of that, I was in a constant state of irritation, which was not a good mental place for me to be. I felt I wasn't being used to the best of my potential, and I couldn't imagine spending the next twenty years in a job where I wasn't allowed to do much.

Later, a different manager took an interest in me and encouraged me to grow. Among other things, she allowed me to take a leadership course. Between that course and my manager's support, I took a fresh look at the work I was doing. I got a lot of support and encouragement from her, but I continued to float down the river—until she left. Then I realized I had no idea what kind of manager I would get next, took control of my rudder, and asked for a job audit. Not only was I granted the audit, but it resulted in my position being upgraded to program coordinator within a couple of months. That was both exciting and unusual because audits had been known to take up to a year to reach resolution. Once again, learning to stand up for myself paid off.

I began my career not knowing my strengths and weaknesses, not knowing how to get clarification about duties and expectations, not knowing that my communication style might confuse others, not understanding that I take things more literally than others, and not knowing that I could stand up for myself. I had to learn a lot on my own, but I also had the support of a few good supervisors.

One experience at the airport highlighted both the challenges and successes for me in my career. I was in a meeting with my supervisor and two coworkers, and during that meeting, I said something my supervisor translated in a way that took the conversation in a different direction than I had intended. I didn't say anything during the meeting, but later, after reorganizing and revaluating the information in my mind, I talked with my supervisor and explained what I had been trying to say. We didn't necessarily agree, but it was clear that we understood each other's position, and that was the point of my asking to speak with my supervisor one-on-one.

The moral of that story is that the person with Turner Syndrome needs to look at body language and listen to the response they get when they're speaking to check if the listener is understanding them. If they think they might have been misunderstood, clarify for the person. And if needed, step back, reevaluate, and go back to the person you were speaking with to make your point another way if it appears you were not understood.

And as a parent of a Turner Syndrome girl, make sure your daughter knows she can reach out to teachers and employers to get clarification on anything from class assignments to job expectations and duties. I wasn't taught that, and it hindered me for a long time.

- **Lesson 1:** *Support your daughter in discovering for herself what she is interested in and has passion for. There are assessment tests that can help with this.*

- **Lesson 2:** *Teach your daughter how to prepare a résumé/ job application and work with her on interview skills, hire someone to do that, or have her school career counselor provide help in these areas.*

- **Lesson 3:** *Encourage your daughter to get clear instructions about job roles and what is expected of* them in their work by communicating with management, seeking ongoing feedback, and making course corrections as necessary. Work is one place where a Turner Syndrome girl cannot be rudderless!

• **Lesson 4:** Teach your daughter to identify and work with the issues that arise with nonverbal learning disorder. Make sure she knows she can and should identify her needs and ask for help when needed.

• **Lesson 5:** Those with TS and NLD may articulate things differently than others and may therefore be misunderstood without knowing that has happened. It is important for them to learn how to read body language, listen for the response from others after they have spoken, and ask questions to make sure they have been understood.

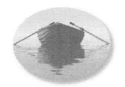

CHAPTER 9

Dealing with Immaturity, Emotions, and Meltdowns

THOSE OF US WITH nonverbal learning disorder tend to be slow in maturing. We have meltdowns just like any regular kid, but we may continue to have meltdowns at twenty, thirty, and older. And meltdowns in adulthood are not only inappropriate, they can be catastrophic in the workplace. They also don't solve whatever problems or issues lead to them.

If you are the parent of a TS girl with nonverbal learning disorder, teach her how to deal with the emotions that trigger meltdowns. When she is little, you can help with a meltdown by talking to her about something other than what is bothering her to divert her mind from the meltdown. Or, as one mother reported in a social media post I saw, you can ask her to sit down and concentrate on her breathing.

Once she's calmer, you can talk with her about what has bothered her. That will help you identify the issue and deal with it. Teach her how to do this on her own: redirect her attention, breathe, calm down, identify the problem, and determine how to deal with the issue. I have one piece of advice on this, though. Don't simply tell her to calm down. No one wants to be told to calm down. It's infuriating because it makes us feel as if our feelings don't matter. Everyone has a right to their feelings. It's just a matter of how we express them and what we do with them.

While we do tend to mature a little slowly, we eventually get there. We need what would be considered normal parameters of behavior explained to us. Since we are behind in maturity and have a tendency to just float down the river, we may not be able to ascertain what is socially acceptable behavior and what is not. What may seem obvious to others is not necessarily obvious to us. Remember the example I gave earlier of a Turner Syndrome girl being asked to take a lipstick sold at a store and put it in her purse? It was shoplifting, but it may not be understood by the girl with Turner Syndrome that it is shoplifting and therefore wrong because we are slow to mature and develop our own internal rudder.

I can count on one hand the times I had meltdowns while growing up. I suppressed the meltdowns, but that didn't mean I was able to suppress the emotions that might have led to them in another girl. I was not taught the correct way to handle my emotions, so I just sucked it up and soldiered on. I have been asked how I feel about specific things and events, and it is a difficult question for me because I didn't learn how to express emotions growing up. Don't get me wrong. I'm a very emotional person when it comes to others and supporting them, but I'm not good at expressing how I feel about things that have to do with me. Someone described me as being an advocate for others. That is true. But those with nonverbal learning disorder don't easily advocate for themselves.

Let me give you an example. Growing up, I had a jewelry box with a few pieces of jewelry in it. A couple of times, my necklaces were missing, and I found them in one or the other of my sister's jewelry boxes. I couldn't name the emotion I felt when I found the jewelry and I certainly couldn't express it. I just took my jewelry back and said nothing.

Most children would confront their sibling and say, "You took my necklaces, and I want them back." They would stand up for themselves. Not only did I not know how to do that, I didn't know I even *could* do that. I just thought that if I had jewelry, it would be taken from me. And it wasn't until I was in my fifties that I realized I could have jewelry and my sisters weren't around to take it from me.

It's important for a girl with Turner Syndrome to learn how to stand up for herself and advocate for herself. And it's important for that girl to know she has the same rights and the same entitlements as anyone else. Teach her about boundaries. Help her build an appropriate sense of self so she has the self-esteem and self-confidence to stand up for herself.

Because a girl with Turner Syndrome may misunderstand what is going on when something happens—like my thinking that jewelry would probably be taken from me—as a parent, you will have to work a little harder than other parents to understand what your daughter is thinking and how she sees the world. Also, some girls with TS who don't know how to translate their emotions may have meltdowns. So you may have to help your daughter learn how to describe what she is feeling and how to express it appropriately.

I wasn't taught those things and have struggled to learn them as an adult. When I went into the hospital for kidney failure, my condo was a mess. Not only did one of my sisters and a niece clean and totally rearrange my condo while I was gone, the same sister also decided my basement storage unit needed to be cleaned out. In that unit, I had around three hundred books stored in plastic tubs to keep them safe from the elements.

Books have always been important to me, both as vehicles for escape and vehicles for collecting information that proves I have intelligence. When my sister said she was going to take the books to a thrift store, I didn't mind so much because I like the idea of paying it forward with books. But when my brother-in-law told me he had actually thrown all of my books away, I was furious. I said nothing because I feared I would be accused of being ungrateful. I also didn't know how to express my emotions effectively, and I didn't know how to advocate for myself.

Your daughter may not be able to completely eliminate meltdowns, but you can help her learn how to avoid them in the first place by helping her learn how to identify and manage her emotions, set appropriate boundaries, and stand up for herself. And when a meltdown does happen, you can help her manage through it.

- **Lesson:** *Just like any child, the girl with TS will need to be taught how to appropriately deal with her emotions. That may require time and patience because those with Turner Syndrome mature a bit more slowly than other girls, may not understand or be able to articulate what they are feeling, may not understand boundaries, and may not have the inner confidence to stand up for themselves.*

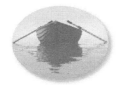

CHAPTER 10

Medical and Other Issues

BEFORE DELVING INTO some of the medical and other issues related to Turner Syndrome, let's talk about the issue of choosing to tell others or not tell others about the condition. To tell or not to tell is an important choice, and it is a choice that may vary depending on circumstances. I tend to not talk about having Turner Syndrome because many people have viewed me differently when I tell them. They then use it as an excuse to treat me as if I have diminished mental capacities or am handicapped. Family did that too. They didn't understand the challenges Turner Syndrome girls have because there was little information about Turner Syndrome at the time. And because they didn't understand the challenges and differences, they didn't accommodate them or help me learn how to manage them. I wasn't even diagnosed with Turner Syndrome until I was seventeen.

All my life I have tried to be as normal as possible, and I have only once used the word "handicapped." Of course, the word "handicapped" is seldom used these days. In business it is more appropriate to ask those with "disabilities" what accommodations they need. I like and agree with that. Can you imagine someone ever asking Steven Hawking, "What's your handicap?" By getting rid of words like "handicapped" or even "disabled," it is easier to focus on what the individual's strengths are instead of their weaknesses.

Those with Turner Syndrome have several medical issues that can be of concern. These are not things to be anxious about, but they do need to be taken into consideration and managed.

The first one is the heart. Usually TS girls have two aortic valve flaps (cusps) instead of the normal three. I am blessed to have three. Those with Turner Syndrome are also more prone to aortic dissection than others. This one is scary because with aortic dissection, the inner layer of the aorta tears. Blood flows through the tear, causing rupturing in the middle and then outer layers of the aorta. This simulates a heart attack, and if the patient is treated like it is a heart attack, the results can be catastrophic and devastating. They may be given medication that will not help the problem when what they need is surgery to repair the tear in the aorta. This is what happened to John Ritter. He was misdiagnosed and died because he didn't receive the correct treatment.

Those with Turner Syndrome may also be born with kidneys that are connected instead of separate, making a U or horseshoe shape. My kidneys are normal, but those with connected kidneys can be prone to kidney stones and urinary tract problems.

Girls with TS also tend to have underactive thyroids. This can create a host of problems. One is sensitivity to temperature. Cold temperatures are difficult for me because I feel the cold more intensely than the average person. An underactive thyroid can also cause weight management issues. We typically carry excess weight. In part, this is caused because an underactive thyroid produces a slower metabolism. But just like anyone else, we need to be taught proper nutrition and the importance of exercise. There are many options for exercise these days. Help your daughter discover one that fits her personality. And don't just assume that excess weight in a TS girl is caused by a lack of good nutrition and a lack of exercise. Managing our weight is more complicated than nutrition and exercise. If the thyroid is underactive, that needs to be managed medically.

We have vision problems. Those with TS are typically myopic. I didn't get a pair of glasses until I was eighteen—just in time for college. Regular eye checkups should be a part of health management for a TS girl and glasses should be provided if needed.

Turner Syndrome also tends to cause bowed arms. My arms curve, so I wear shirts with long sleeves. I try to hide my arms because I'm embarrassed by them. When I was in kindergarten, one of my sisters had just learned first aid at school and tried to practice on me by splinting my arm. Of course, it didn't work because my arm was bowed and wouldn't conform to her splint. But I didn't realize my arms were different at the time, and when I did, I was embarrassed about them.

Higher than normal liver enzymes are another TS symptom, and it is one I have. It is caused by fatty liver, which is normal for those with TS. Unfortunately, none of the doctors I went to connected my fatty liver to having Turner Syndrome because they were largely uneducated about TS. And it wasn't until I attended a Turner Syndrome conference a couple of years ago that I learned coffee has the potential to elevate liver enzymes. Since then, I have cut down on my coffee intake. These days, there are supplements and treatment approaches that help with liver issues, and your daughter's doctor can help.

Because of our weight and liver issues, TS girls are prone to diabetes. Make sure her doctor knows this and monitors her for this potential issue. If your daughter does have diabetes, there are many ways to help control and manage it. Again, your daughter's physician can guide you on this.

Lymphedema is another potential challenge with TS girls. It most often causes swelling in our extremities—our hands and feet. I once saw a picture of me and my mom right after my birth. I was a little puff ball. That is common with TS and is often the first signal that something is genetically wrong. Throughout my life, I have noticed that my hands and feet swell slightly every once in a while. It's not enough for radical adjustments in my case, but it can be for some TS women.

There is a potential for dental issues, including issues with tooth, root, and facial bone development. I don't particularly have dental issues but have been told I have a high arch to the roof of my mouth. Make sure your daughter sees a dentist as early as possible after the diagnosis of Turner Syndrome to assess whether she has any dental issues related to TS.

We are also prone to osteoporosis, and I have been diagnosed with this. Speak with your doctor about options for treating it. Bone density and bone health are related to the hormones generated during menstrual cycles, and while young women may not give this much thought, it can be an issue later in life. No one wants osteoporosis or osteopenia, which is what can happen with age. Regardless of age, there has to be a balance of hormones for health. But girls with Turner Syndrome usually have nonfunctioning ovaries, which means they do not begin producing estrogen or progesterone at puberty. Not only does the lack of functioning ovaries mean that the TS girl will be infertile, it also means that without medical hormone treatment, they will not have the usual sex hormones so important to health.

As I stated earlier, I was not diagnosed with TS until I was seventeen and didn't have any kind of hormone therapy until I was nineteen. At nineteen, I was given two pills to stimulate a menstrual cycle. But because of their cost and the fact I generally didn't like having periods, I didn't routinely take them. Then, when I was in my early thirties, my gynecologist told me something that changed how serious I was about taking my hormone replacement pills. He told me I was at a greater risk for cancer if I didn't have periods, and one of the forms of cancer for which I would be more at risk was uterine cancer. That got my attention because from what we were able to piece together, my grandmother on my father's side died of uterine cancer. Talk about putting the fear of God into someone! That doctor prescribed birth control pills for me, so I only had the expense of one prescription. I started taking them routinely from then on. And I began noticing the kind of physical changes that usually happen to girls when they reach puberty.

TS girls can have a webbed neck. This is what is known as the linebacker neck. It can be corrected with surgery. I don't have this attribute, but I do have a short, thick neck. For that reason, I'm conscious about necklines on blouses as well as how necklaces and scarves frame my neck.

We typically do not grow very tall. Growth hormone is now an option. It wasn't when I was growing up because it was still considered experimental. I was given testosterone for a couple of years, and I did grow two inches taller. Today, there are many options for growth hormone, and it is advantageous for the parent of a TS girl to discuss them with their pediatrician and then with their daughter when she starts questioning her small stature. It's her body, and she needs to have input into treatment.

There are often issues with depression and anxiety in those with TS. I have been fortunate. The only time depression was an issue for me was when I was working for a temp agency and had no insurance. I was making too little money to consider seeing a doctor, so I was not able to get a prescription for the thyroid medication I needed. And no one told me that not having my thyroid meds would make me as depressed as I got. Fortunately, a coworker told me about a clinic for low-income individuals, and I finally saw a doctor. I was able to get my meds and got back on track.

Anxiety does plague me. It's why I have cats and read so much. Cats keep me calm. Loving them and taking care of them just plain makes me feel good. Of course, it helps that they return the unconditional love you give them. And reading gives my mind something to do besides mulling over things that might cause worry.

I also have a tendency to generalize, which can add to the issue with anxiety. For example, for several Christmases, I made little goodie bags for my family because I couldn't afford presents of any other kind for everyone. The goody bags consisted of candy canes, nuts, hot chocolate, and two types of mincemeat tarts I had made. After one Christmas, one of my sisters told me that my efforts were not appreciated. I believed she was speaking for the whole family, so I never made the goody bags again. I generalized what she said.

Decision-making can also be a problem. We can reach the same conclusion as someone who does not have Turner Syndrome, but it takes us longer because of the way we're hardwired. As children, we need a little more help in learning how to make decisions than others so we can really get the decision-making process down, and like other children, we need to be included in decisions that affect us. When we ask questions, we are not necessarily questioning your decision, we are simply trying to figure how you arrived at your conclusion so we can process it in a manner we can understand.

Whatever life throws at your TS daughter can be handled with a combination of patience, love, medical attention, strategies to help with cognitive issues, and doses of understanding. There are many more resources now than there were when I was young. Take advantage of them. Current resources include the Turner Syndrome Society of the United States, Turner clinics, and local TS organizations that help you to connect to local resources. Don't allow yourself or your daughter to become discouraged. Help is out there and available.

- **Lesson:** *Take one issue at a time. Each child will have their own unique issues. Take a deep breath and deal with what has been given to you and your daughter.*

CHAPTER 11

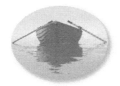

I'm Just Me

WHILE IT IS TRUE that girls with Turner Syndrome and nonverbal learning disorder have some challenges, like everyone else, they also have strengths. We want to be treated as individuals and not simply classified as TS/NLD girls and women. I want to be treated as just me, the same way you are treated as just you, with differences that encompass strengths and weakness on an individual basis. I want to learn about my uniqueness and how to leverage my strengths and cope with my weaknesses like anyone else. And while those of us with Turner Syndrome have some differences that come with the condition, one of the main ones is that we require more patience and repetition due to the way we process information. So don't give up on us. Just take a deep breath and lather, rinse, and repeat.

Acknowledgments

I WISH TO THANK Dr. Dean Mooney of the Maple Leaf Clinic in Vermont for his support, time, and input into this project. I also wish to thank the Turner Syndrome Society of the United States (TSSUS) for teaching me about Turner Syndrome and generally helping me to accept myself for who I am.

About the Author

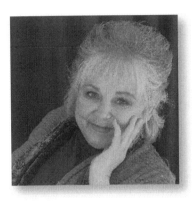

MARY YOAKUM knows a little about Turner Syndrome and nonverbal learning disorder because she has lived her life with these conditions and has made a study of them. Through her personal experience, she has learned a few lessons she would like to share with others. Mary is now retired from working at Denver International Airport and lives with her two cats, Otis and Sally, in Denver, Colorado. She enjoys going to museums, attending church, and volunteering at the library.